ACID
REFLUX
DIET

101 Best Foods
To Treat & Cure GERD

Health Research Staff

Published by:

Millwood Media
PO Box 1220
Melrose, FL 32666 USA

www.MillwoodMediaEpub.com

ISBN 13: 978-1-937918-72-9

Health Disclaimer

Any and all information contained herein is not intended to take the place of medical advice from a health care professional. Any action taken based on these contents is at the sole discretion and sole liability of the reader.

Readers should always consult appropriate health professionals on any matter relating to their health and well-being before taking any action of any kind concerning health-related issues. Any information or opinions provided here or in any Millwood Media related articles, materials or information are believed to be accurate and sound, however Millwood Media assumes no liability for the use or misuse of information provided by Millwood Media.

No personnel or associates of Millwood Media will in any way be held responsible by any reader who fails to consult the appropriate health authorities with respect to their individual health care before acting on or using any information contained herein, and neither the author or publisher of any of this information will be held responsible for errors or omissions, or use or misuse of the information.

Urgent Plea!

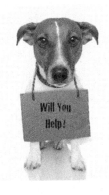

Thank you for buying my bosses' book! It will really help life around here. Would you please help our Health Research Staff (and me) and go back to the site where you purchased this book and leave your feedback. They need your feedback to make the next version better. Arf! Arf!

Contents

Contents

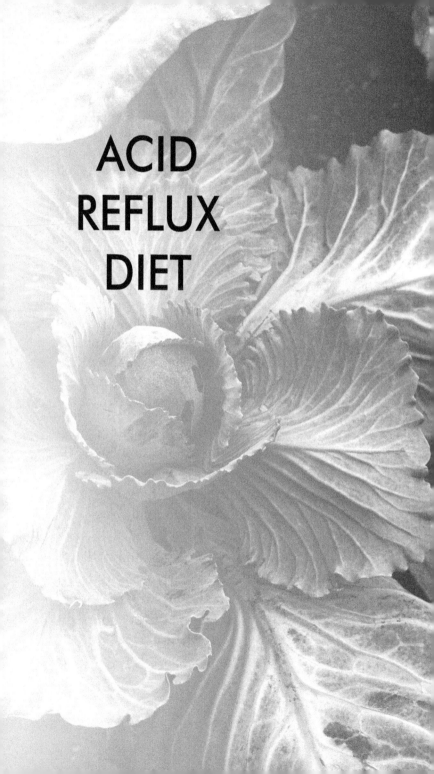

ACID
REFLUX
DIET

INTRODUCTION

If you're someone who is suffering from Gastroesophageal reflux disease, otherwise referred to as GERD for short, you know just how painful and aggravating this condition can be.

This is a quite common disorder that many people suffer from and comes about when the stomach acid refluxes into the lower esophagus region through the lower esophageal sphincter. When this is occurring, there is a backflow of the stomach's contents into the esophagus, which then can cause a a few negative symptoms to occur.

The two primary common side effects present in those who are suffering from GERD include:

- Persistent heartburn that never seems to let up

- A burning feeling of discomfort in the upper chest as well as abdomen

For some people this occurs only after eating a meal and on an occasional basis, while for others it's present each and every time they eat a meal and tends to last much longer in duration.

Typically the underlying conditions that tend to bring on GERD include a lower pressure level in the lower esophageal sphincter, irritation of the lining of the esophagus, which is typically brought on by the diet, along with an improper clearance of the esophageal acid from the area.

In addition to this, some people will also notice delayed stomach emptying, so that too can be a reason why you may start to experience pain and discomfort associated with the condition.

The most common factors that can cause one to develop GERD include lifestyle and dietary choices, which is good news because it means the condition can be treated quite well as long as you are willing to make some pivotal changes to your everyday habits.

The most problematic foods that need to be avoided are chocolate, peppermint, fried or very fatty foods, coffee and alcohol beverages.

Those who are suffering are instructed to try and limit their consumption of acidic foods, eating more alkaline foods instead, while keeping high fat meat and dairy products out of the picture.

By transitioning over to a diet that's filled with the proper foods and focusing on eating slightly smaller meals more frequently throughout the day to reduce the amount of stress that's placed on the system, you can effectively control and combat GERD.

In this book, we're going to cover all the main foods that you should be eating in your diet to effectively help treat the condition and free yourself from GERD symptoms for the time to come.

If you stay consistent with your efforts and make sure that you are not letting the wrong foods enter your system, you should start to see significant improvements almost immediately.

Let's take a look at the top 101 foods for GERD that you need to know.

Attention All Eagle Eyes: We've had a number of people proof this book before we released it to you, but there is a chance you might spot something that was missed. If you find a typo or other obvious error please send it to us. And if you're the first one to report it, we'll send you a free gift! Send to: millwoodmedia@gmail.com

---

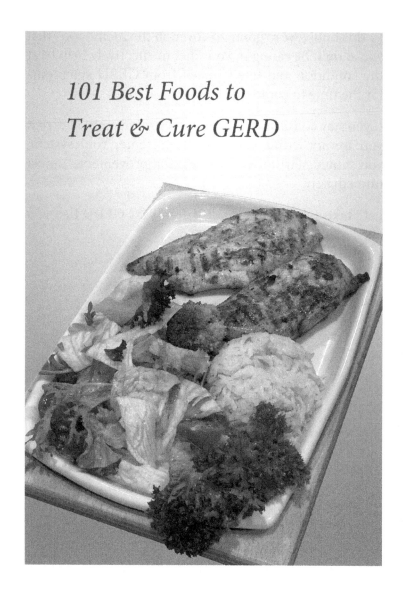

101 Best Foods to Treat & Cure GERD

1. ACAI BERRY

This fruit has been talked about a great deal in the media for the wide number of benefits it's supposed to offer. First, it's jam packed with antioxidants that will help to fend off free radical damage. In addition to that, it also contains a number of important minerals and vitamins as well as omega fatty acids, which is rare for a fruit to contain. This fruit is rich in potassium, manganese, copper, iron, and magnesium. While the jury is still out as to whether it qualifies as a true superfood, it has been shown to offer help to those with GERD. Make sure that you don't overlook adding it to your diet plan.

2. ALFALFA

Alfalfa sprouts are a low-calorie, nutritious food to add to your diet and are rich in vitamin A, niacin, calcium, as well as dietary fiber. In addition to that, they're also full of vitamin C, vitamin K, thiamin, riboflavin, along with folate, so will provide the body with many nutrients to support optimal function. Aflafla sprouts can help to boost your immune system due to their vitamin A and C combination and work great in sandwiches, salads, or placed into a whole wheat pita.

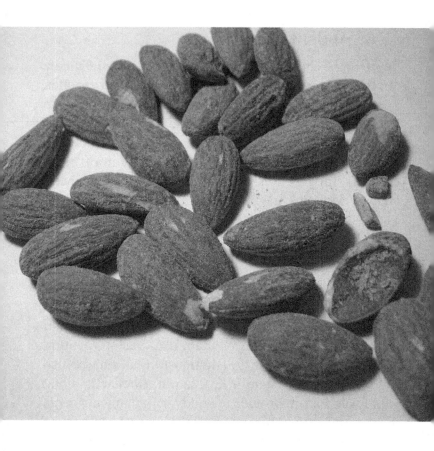

3. ALMONDS

Almonds are one of the most commonly consumed nut varieties and are a great addition to any GERD diet plan. They're an alkaline based food, so won't increase your risk for stomach acid development and add a nice mild flavor to the dishes that you're preparing. Almonds are high in manganese, rich in vitamin E, high in magnesium, and a good source of tryptophan, copper, vitamin B2, and phosphorus. They are higher in calories however due to their healthy fat content, so just be sure that you are eating them in moderation and controlling your portion size. Those suffering from GERD do want to consume smaller, less calorie dense meals, so take caution to only eat about an ounce.

4. ALMOND BUTTER

Almond butter is a great addition to your diet as a condiment to replace regular butter and is full of healthy fats along with some muscle building protein. Almond butter offers a nice change of pace compared to regular peanut butter and gives a creamy taste to any dish you serve it with. Almond butter contains similar nutrients to that of regular almonds including magnesium, manganese, copper, phosphorus, and vitamin B2. Just like with almonds, watch how much you are eating to keep your calorie count under control. Serve it smeared over an apple, on a slice of whole grain bread, or mix it into a protein shake.

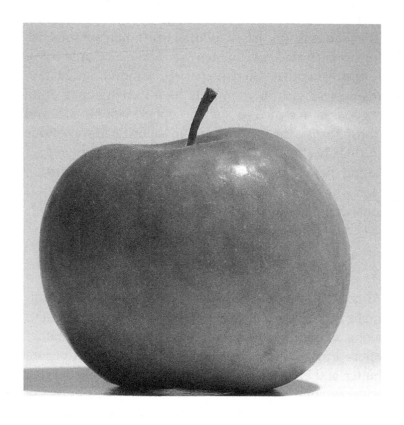

5. ALMOND MILK

If you're someone who loves milk but can't deal with lactose, a good alternative for you may be almond milk. This one is also a great choice for anyone suffering from GERD as it will help to ease your symptoms quite nicely. In addition to that, it's high in vitamin E, manganese, phosphorus, potassium, selenium, iron, fiber, zinc, and calcium, but yet is much lower in calories than regular milk, coming in at only 40 calories per one cup serving. Regular skim milk contains 91, so it can add up if you drink multiple glasses of milk daily. Since almond milk contains no saturated fats, this also makes it a great addition for anyone suffering from heart burn.

6. APPLES

One of the best fruits to eat for those who are suffering from GERD is the apple. Apples come in many different varieties and are a great way to add more dietary fiber to your day. Apples contain certain enzymes that help assist with the breakdown of carbohydrates in the body and may assist with blood sugar control when eating them regularly. In addition to that, those who eat apples on a regular basis tend to report feeling more satisfied with their diet overall, so this may be a great way to keep your calorie intake in check and experience an easier time maintaining your body weight. Try apples alone, chopped into a salad, baked with your main protein source, or cut into a fruit salad.

7. APPLESAUCE, UNSWEETENED

Applesauce is a nice addition to your diet plan if you aren't in the mood for a whole apple or are preparing baked goods that require additional moisture. You can easily replace some of the oil in your baking for applesauce instead, making those foods more GERD-friendly. Applesauce contains a good dose of vitamin C and will also provide some dietary fiber, just as whole apples would. At just over 100 calories per one cup serving, it's a smart addition to any diet plan. If eating it plain, try it with a little cinnamon on top for added flavor.

8. APRICOTS

Apricots are a small fruit that serve as a quick snack any time and are relatively low in calories. They are going to provide you with vitamin A, which is great for protecting your eyes and strengthening the immune system along with some vitamin C as well, helping to offer antioxidant support. Apricots can be added to many different dishes such as to your morning bowl of cereal, to some oatmeal pancakes you're preparing, or on top of baked or grilled chicken dishes. They also work terrific in salads or mixed into a fruit salad. Offering a few grams of fiber, this is also a good food for decreasing your hunger level.

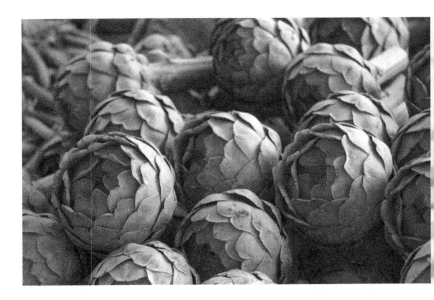

9. ARTICHOKES

The artichoke is an often overlooked vegetable that offers numerous health benefits, so you should start reconsidering adding it to your diet plan. This vegetable is rich in vitamin C, vitamin B, and will provide some vitamin K to support good blood clotting abilities as well. In addition to that, artichokes are also high in copper, calcium, potassium, and iron, so will support higher energy levels as you go about your day. Those who aren't getting in enough iron often fall prey to fatigue, so it's essential that you are taking steps to meet your daily requirements. Try artichokes boiled or barbequed for great flavor.

10. ASPARAGUS

Asparagus is a nutrient rich vegetable that especially stands out for its vitamin K content. In addition to this vitamin, it'll also provide vitamin A, folate, iron, vitamin B1, vitamin C, tryptophan, vitamin B2, fiber, and manganese. Asparagus is going to help to reduce the level of inflammation in the body while upping your antioxidant protection to help defend against invading free radicals that may be attacking. This vegetable is great for boosting your digestive health as well due to a particular nutrient it contains called inulin. Finally, asparagus packs in a good dose of fiber at 3 grams per cup and will also provide 4-5 grams of protein. For anyone who struggles to meet their protein and fiber needs, this is a must-have food to add to your diet plan and can help to increase the passage of starch through your system, as noted in a study published in the British Journal of Nutrition.

11. AVOCADO

Avocados are a unique fruit because of the fact that they contain healthy fats, so they'll not only provide good antioxidant support like most fruits do, but also help to control and regulate blood sugar levels as you won't get nearly the same degree of blood glucose spike from consuming them. Avocados contain phytosterols, which can help to reduce the level of inflammation in the body and treat pain and discomfort associated with arthritis. In addition to that, they also support heart health and can reduce your risk of developing cancer. Serve them in sandwiches, salads, as a dip, or simply on the side of your meal for a creamy taste that's sure to satisfy.

12. BANANAS

Bananas are a great fruit to eat for anyone leading an active lifestyle due to their high potassium content, as well as starch that will provide your muscles usable energy quickly. Bananas are a very alkaline fruit, so they won't cause issues with stomach acid, and are especially helpful in treating those who are suffering from GERD. Bananas are also rich in vitamin B6 as well as vitamin C and can help to balance out the electrolyte levels in the body, assisting anyone who is suffering from problems with elimination. Bananas are also great for those who are worried about or suffering from stomach ulcers, as they help to eliminate bacteria in the stomach that can cause these problems. Bananas, with their high potassium level and dietary fiber content, are also going to be good for those who are trying to boost their heart health. Try bananas topped over your morning bowl of cereal, added to a fruit smoothie, eaten with some almond butter, or just served up on their own for a fast boost of energy any time you need it.

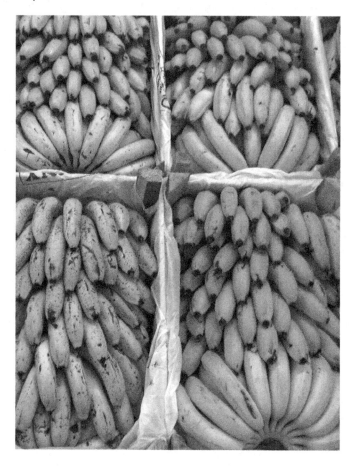

13. BASIL

Basil is a great way to flavor your food if you're suffering from GERD, and won't add any calories or fat to your dish. This spice is going to rank in high for its vitamin K content, so it is good for helping to ensure that your blood is able to clot properly. Basil contains eugenol which helps to reduce the level of inflammation that occurs in the body, so it can be a great addition to the diet if you're suffering from health concerns such as rheumatoid arthritis or inflammatory bowel conditions. It also has strong antioxidant-like properties as noted by a study in the Journal of Agriculture Food Chemistry. Finally, it may also help to boost your cardiovascular health, so that's just one more reason to make sure that you are adding it to your diet regularly. Try it sprinkled over pasta, added to salads, or used on any lean meat sources you're preparing.

14. BEEF, GROUND, EXTRA LEAN

When on a GERD diet, it's important that you're limiting your intake of fats, so choosing extra lean beef is a must. When chosen wisely, extra lean ground beef can be a good addition to your diet because it's high in protein content, rich in iron, and a good source of zinc, vitamin B3, vitamin B6, and vitamin B12. For anyone who is looking to build some lean muscle mass, this nutrient combination is perfect. Extra lean ground beef can be used to prepare meatballs or home-made hamburgers, and you can use oatmeal in replacement of bread crumbs. Just be sure to run hot water over the beef after it's finished cooking, as this will help to eliminate much of the fat content as well.

15. BEETS

Beets are a fantastic food for providing health benefits to the body as they'll help to boost your antioxidant support, decrease the level of inflammation present in your tissues, and can also help to provide detoxification benefits. Yet, few people ever make use of these with their diet plan. Beets will provide you with folate, manganese, fiber and potassium, so they can also help to keep your energy levels high. Finally, the fiber variety found in beets may be especially good for boosting your digestive tract health and preventing prostate cancer, as noted by a study in the Cancer Epidemiol Biomarkers Prevention journal, so for anyone suffering from digestive concerns or at risk for this variation of cancer, beets are a great addition to their plan. Serve them on their own or add them into salad or soup instead.

16. BLACKBERRIES

Blackberries are a tasty fruit to add to your diet that will pack in additional nutrients and are also high in antioxidants, vitamin E, folate, magnesium, potassium, copper, vitamin K, vitamin C, and manganese. Blackberries also contain a very strong dose of fiber, so are good for helping to regulate your blood glucose levels, decreasing your risk of developing diabetes over the long term, while also helping to keep your energy level on a more even keel. Blackberries can be eaten on their own, tossed into a bowl of cereal, added to a fruit smoothie, or served with some yogurt instead.

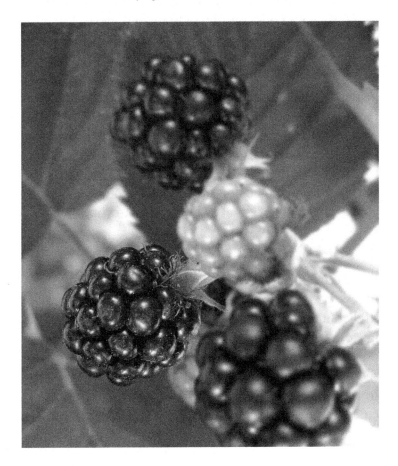

17. BLACK BEANS

Black beans are a terrific source of fiber, so they can help to boost your digestive track health and promote better regularity. Black beans are a very good food for anyone suffering from GERD to consider adding to their diet because of the fact that they will provide protein and help to reduce your consumption of higher fat meat sources in your diet. Remember that it's a must that you are limiting how much saturated fat you eat, and since black beans are free from saturated fat, this makes them a top pick. Black beans can also help to enhance your overall blood glucose control because they contain complex carbohydrates, which break down slowly in the body, so will release a steady stream of energy over time. Finally, adding beans to your diet can help to lower your risk of heart disease or other heart related conditions. So if you're suffering or are at risk, they're a great food to add into your diet.

18. BLACK CURRENT

Black currents are a fruit that many people overlook entirely but that do really have a lot to offer from a nutritional point of view. They're the second highest fruit for both iron and protein, two nutrients that most fruits lack, so if you're struggling to meet your

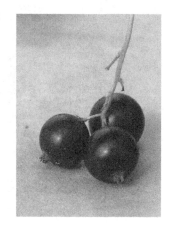

intake, they are a smart addition to your diet. They also contain five times the amount of vitamin C that you get from oranges, so are great for those looking to enhance their immune system as well. In addition to that, they also pack in some calcium, so they earn top marks for promoting bone health. If you eat the seeds, you'll also take in the extremely important omega acids.

19. BLUEBERRIES

Well known for their antioxidant content, blueberries are a good addition to your GERD diet plan. Blueberries contain certain antioxidants that are especially important for promoting good brain health, so can help to increase your focus and concentration levels. In addition to that, they'll also strengthen your nervous system and reduce the amount of oxidative stress you suffer from. Blueberries are also good for regulating your blood glucose levels, so may assist with controlling energy and preventing diabetes. Try adding some to your yogurt or favorite muffin mix.

20. BOK CHOY

Bok Choy can be a great addition to your diet plan and serve as a replacement for other lettuce varieties that you might be consuming. It contains just 13 calories per one cup serving so won't hardly add any energy value to your menu, making it ideal for those seeking weight control. In addition to that, it's also rich in vitamin C, high in vitamin K, and provides a number of important B vitamins that are required to support a healthy metabolic rate and strong energy levels. Finally, it'll provide some bone boosting calcium and phosphorus, along with potassium, manganese, and iron to keep your energy levels strong.

21. BROCCOLI

A fantastic food to help lower your cholesterol levels and boost heart health, broccoli is also great for defending against cancer. This food is going to help to detoxify the body, offering cleansing benefits that will get you feeling your best on a daily basis. It contains a number of important nutrients including vitamin C, vitamin K, folate, vitamin A, manganese, fiber, as well as potassium, vitamin B6, vitamin B2, phosphorus, and magnesium. Broccoli works great eaten raw with a low fat dip, added to salads, stir-fried, baked, or steamed. It's a very versatile vegetable that most people do enjoy.

22. BRUSSELS SPROUTS

Brussels sprouts often have people turning their nose up, but they really do offer serious nutrition that you shouldn't take lightly. This vegetable packs in a potent dose of vitamin K, vitamin C, manganese, as well as folate, vitamin A, potassium, B vitamins, phosphorus, and iron. In addition to that, it's high in calcium content, so can help to promote stronger bones. This food is great for reducing the amount of chronic oxidative stress in the body, so it can help to treat a wide variety of conditions including the prevention of cancer. Try them steamed for best health benefits.

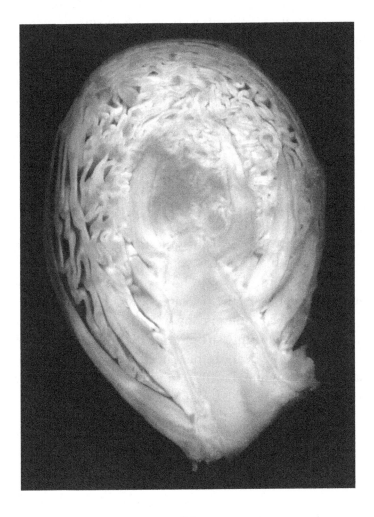

23. BUCKWHEAT

Buckwheat is a great high energy food to add to your diet to help boost your energy levels while controlling your blood sugar. It's a great source of manganese, tryptophan and magnesium, and will also provide plenty of dietary fiber to help keep your blood sugar levels stabilized, and your energy on an even keel. In addition to that, buckwheat can help to boost your cardiovascular system and lower your risk of developing diabetes. This grain can also help to reduce your risk of developing gallstones, so it can help to improve your intestinal system's health overall. Finally, it contains key lignans that can slash your risk of developing heart disease.

24. BRAN CEREAL

Bran is a good food to consume in your diet regularly if you're looking to boost your fiber consumption. It's typically quite low in sugar, however be sure to read the nutritional label on the package as this isn't always the case. Also, check sodium content to be sure that the bran cereal you're selecting isn't ranking high for this mineral. All in all, bran cereal can be a healthy way to start your day when combined with skim or almond milk, and some fresh berries or a banana on top.

25. BUTTER LETTUCE

Butter lettuce is a food that's low in calories, and makes for a great substitute in your diet plan for the regular lettuce varieties that you might be eating. This lettuce variety is high in thiamin, riboflavin, calcium, magnesium, phosphorus, and will even supply some vitamin C, vitamin A, vitamin B6, folate, iron, potassium, and manganese. Serve it up in any salad you're preparing, or have it in a sandwich with whatever other vegetables you're consuming with it.

26. CABBAGE

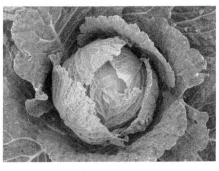

Cabbage is a fantastic vegetable for offering strong antioxidant and cancer protection that is also very low in calories, so it's ideal for those who are watching their weight. Cabbage is rich in vitamin K, vitamin C, folate, manganese, vitamin B6, potassium, tryptophan, and will even provide a small dose of calcium to help promote strong bones. Cabbage can assist with reducing the amount of inflammation present in the body and may also assist with reducing your risk of developing cancer. It works great in salads, stir-fries, baked, or prepared in soup.

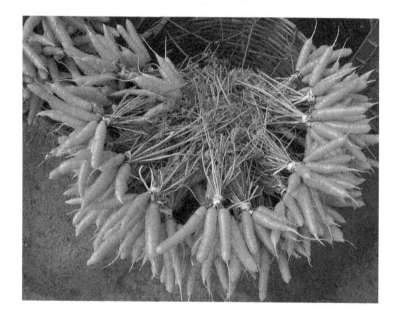

27. CANTALOUPE

For a sweet treat anytime, consider serving up some cantaloupe. This melon is low in calories, at just 50 calories or so per cup, and will pack in plenty of good nutrition. It's going to provide you with well over 100% of your total daily vitamin C needs, as well as 120% of your vitamin A needs, making it incredibly good for top notch antioxidant support. It's also going to supply you with a good dose of niacin, vitamin B6, folate and potassium, so it is a great choice for anyone involved in a higher intensity exercise program. It also contains no cholesterol, so it will be good for those who are looking to boost their overall heart health.

28. CARROTS

Carrots are a sweeter tasting vegetable that are sure to please almost anyone, even the fussiest of eaters, so they are a great way to increase your total vegetable consumption for the day. Carrots are going to provide plenty of vitamin A, vitamin K, fiber, vitamin C, potassium, as well as many of the B vitamins needed to support a properly functioning metabolism. Carrots rank in high for their antioxidant content and will help to defend against free radical damage, while also boosting your cardiovascular health. Regular consumption of carrots shows a decreased risk of cardiovascular disease development.

29. CAYENNE PEPPER

Cayenne pepper is a great way to add more flavor to your foods, and they help to reduce the heart burn and acid reflux that you may be experiencing. While some people may worry the spice will do the opposite, it really does earn top marks to assist those who are suffering with this condition. Cayenne pepper is a good source of vitamin A, vitamin E, vitamin C, and will also even supply a small dose of calories. Best of all, there are certain compounds in cayenne pepper that will increase your basal metabolic rate, helping you burn calories faster for hours after you consume it. For this reason, it's a perfect addition to anyone's diet who's hoping to achieve optimal weight loss success.

30. CELERY

Celery is a terrific food that's rich in vitamin K, folate, and vitamin A, and contains hardly any calories at all so you can virtually eat as much of it as you want without worry. Celery can help to reduce the amount of blood pressure you experience, and also acts as a diuretic in the body. So if you're retaining water for whatever reason, it's a great treatment for that. Eating celery on a regular basis may also help to lower the level of cholesterol you have in the body, and acts as a 'filler' in your meals, allowing you to eat more bulk without upping the calorie content. Try celery in stir-fry's, soups, salads, or even eaten raw with a little almond butter for a quick snack anytime.

31. CHAMOMILE TEA

Chamomile tea can be a great way to calm symptoms associated with GERD, and is also often used to treat insomnia, anxiety and panic attacks, stomach flu's, and even menstrual cramps. It provides a very soothing feel, so is the perfect way to end a stressful day. Just be sure to serve yours up without the addition of sugar to keep it promoting overall good health.

32. CHERRIES

Cherries are a delicious fruit that's available during the warmer summer months, and pack in sound nutrition as well. They'll offer a good dose of vitamin C, vitamin A, and supply a small amount of calcium and iron as well. Cherries are also a source of natural melatonin, which is a hormone that's produced naturally in the body that helps to regulate your sleeping and waking cycles. By making sure that cherries are included in your diet, you'll find that you fall asleep faster and have better quality sleep once you are sleeping.

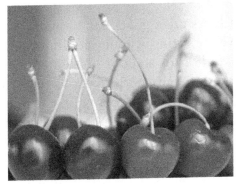

33. CHICKEN BREAST, SKINLESS

Chicken breast meat is a common staple in many diet plans, due to its high protein nature and the fact that it's lower in fat than many other protein rich foods. For those suffering from GERD, it's also good because of the fact it does contain much less saturated fat. Chicken is a great source of tryptophan, as it'll supply you with 128% of your total daily recommended intake. In addition to that, it's also a great source of vitamin B3, selenium, vitamin B6, phosphorus, and choline. The nutrient combination it offers makes it a good choice to help reduce your risk of cancer, and it can also help to lower the risk of mental decline that occurs naturally with age. Finally, with the high B vitamin content, it'll also work very well to keep your energy levels higher, so you can maintain the active lifestyle you enjoy.

34. CHIVES

Chives are a good way to boost the flavor of the meals you're eating without adding any calories at all, or the addition of sodium or saturated fat. While chives are pretty much calorie free (or so close to it you can consider them to be), this does not mean they don't come without a great nutritional punch. Chives are rich in thiamin, niacin, pantothenic acid, phosphorus, zinc, as well as vitamin A, vitamin C, vitamin K, riboflavin, vitamin B6, folate, calcium, iron, magnesium, potassium, and copper. They will provide good support for maintaining a strong immune system, along with ensuring that you are maintaining high energy levels, as you go about any physical activity you perform. Try serving them up on a baked sweet potato, tossed over fish, in a salad, or in any other dish you feel they would work well in.

35. CILANTRO

Cilantro is another great spice that you can safely add to your GERD diet plan to boost the flavor of your foods, without having to turn to condiments high in saturated fat. Cilantro works great served along with a salad dressing as well, so you may consider mixing it right into the ingredients as you prepare your own home-made variety. It's a spice that packs in good nutrition, being rich in niacin, vitamin B6, phosphorus, zinc, selenium, as well as vitamin A, vitamin C, vitamin K, thiamin, riboflavin, folate, calcium, iron, magnesium, potassium, and manganese. The vitamin C content in this spice will also serve as an antioxidant in the body, reducing the chances that you suffer from the damaging effects of free radicals.

36. COCONUT

Coconut is a unique fat in that it's a form of saturated fat, so while you may think it's an unhealthy choice, the truth is that it isn't. This fat variety is referred to as a medium chain triglyceride, which means that it can actually be broken down and used readily by the body as a primary energy source. For those who are reducing the carbohydrate content of their diet, this is a huge benefit that cannot go overlooked. In addition to that, coconut can help to improve your cholesterol profile, reducing your risk of heart disease. Coconut has a great balance of electrolytes as well, with more and more people adding coconut water to their day after intense workout sessions. Coconut may also help to reduce the level of inflammation in the body and will assist with the process of digestion. Finally, it does contain some important fatty acids including lauric acid, caprylic acid, and capric acid, all of which can further reduce inflammation levels in the body. Try some coconut oil drizzled over a salad or add unsweetened dried coconut to baked goods or even into a protein shake for something completely different.

37. COD

Cod is one of the lower fat fish varieties with just 2 grams per 231 gram serving, and will also pack in plenty of protein, giving you 41 grams total for the same serving size. Cod is rich in vitamin D, so it can assist with bone growth and development, and is also a great source of niacin, vitamin B6, vitamin B12, potassium, and selenium. Those who eat fresh fish on a daily basis tend to show decreased rates of heart disease, so it's definitely one food that you want to consider adding to your regular diet plan.

38. CORN BRAN CEREAL

Corn bran cereal is a good complex carbohydrate to consider adding to your GERD diet plan. This cereal is well tolerated by most people and, as long as you select a lower sugar variety, will produce a reliable source of energy that lasts for hours after consuming it. Corn bran cereal will also provide a good dose of dietary fiber, helping to slow the release of the carbohydrates in the blood stream and helping to boost heart health while decreasing your overall cholesterol level. Serve it up with some skim milk (or almond milk if you prefer not to drink dairy).

39. CREAM CHEESE, FAT FREE

Most people regard cream cheese as a high fat condiment, but if you choose the fat free variety, this can be a good addition to your diet plan. The nice thing about fat free cream cheese is that it is low in calories, coming in around only 20 per tablespoon serving, and will provide a small dose of protein as well. For anyone who loves cheesecake, this product makes it perfectly possible to add that to your diet plan on occasion. Cream cheese will also offer a small dose of calcium to help promote healthier bones. Try some on a whole grain bagel, served with salmon, or placed into a stem of celery if you're craving something crunchy.

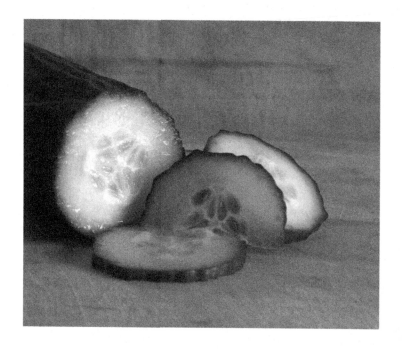

40. CUCUMBER

Cucumbers are a vegetable with a very mild taste so are typically enjoyed by most people. In addition, they are great added to salads or simply eaten on their own. This vegetable contains a number of flavonoids and ligans, along with phytonutrients that will offer clear antioxidant support and assist you with defending against free radical damage. Cucumbers can help to reduce the level of inflammation in the body, as mentioned in a study published in the Current Pharmaceutical Design journal, and also reduce your risk of developing cancer. They're rich in vitamin K content and also provide a small dose of vitamin C, potassium, magnesium, and tryptophan. Add some to the next salad that you eat.

41. ENDIVE

Endive is a great lettuce variety to replace your standard choice with for something completely unique and different, offering you the change in your diet that you crave. This food is very low in calories with just 87 per head, and is virtually fat free. It also contains a potent dose of dietary fiber, at 16 grams per one head serving, and will supply you with a quarter of your daily iron requirements. It's also rich in vitamin A, supplying over 200% of your recommended daily intake and will provide some vitamin C, calcium, vitamin K, thiamin, riboflavin, folate, and zinc as well. For anyone who enjoys salads as a regular part of their diet plan, this is a must-have food.

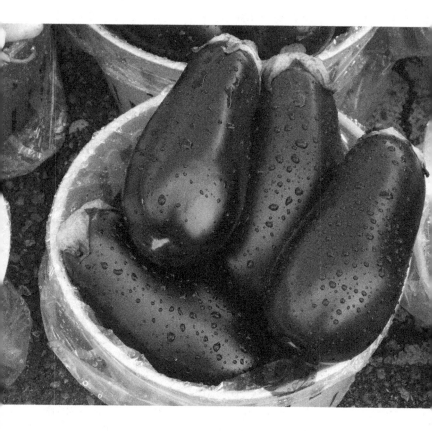

42. EGGPLANT

Eggplant is a vegetable that offers strong benefits for your mind, as it'll help to reduce the chances that your brain is impacted with free radical damage. With strong antioxidant support from eggplant, your entire body will function better, as you feel far healthier on a day to day basis when it's consumed regularly. This vegetable is also high in phenolic antioxidant compounds, which will help to reduce the level of oxidative stress taking place. Finally, it'll boost cardiovascular health by improving blood flow to and from the heart, while reducing the level of bad cholesterol in the blood. Try it baked with other vegetables or as part of a stir-fry.

43. EGG WHITES

Egg whites are very often the primary choice by those who are watching their body weight, as they allow you to get in a terrific source of protein without the regular fat that eggs provide. Egg whites are essentially fat free, and pack in over 4 grams per egg white along with other important nutrients such as selenium, vitamin B6, vitamin D, and vitamin B12. These are all important for maintaining high energy levels in the body and promoting the process of cell growth and division. Try egg whites scrambled or prepared into an omelette and topped with fresh chives or home-made fruit salsa. Just keep in mind that they are slightly higher in sodium, so you should limit yourself to a few each day for optimal health benefits.

44. FETA CHEESE, LOW FAT

Feta cheese is a delicious form of cheese that many people enjoy, and when you choose the lower fat varieties, it can be part of a healthy GERD diet plan. This cheese works great in salads, or topped over whole grain pasta, and will offer a good dose of protein along with calcium. Those who consume more calcium in their diet plan will have an easier time achieving overall fat loss, particularly abdominal fat loss, so it's a cheese variety that you should consider.

45. FIGS

Figs are a good food to be adding to your diet plan due to their high potassium content, which can help to assist with the lowering of blood pressure levels, as proven by a study in the New England Journal of Medicine. In addition to that, figs are also high in dietary fiber, so they can help to lower the overall amount of cholesterol in the blood, promoting better heart health for you overall. Furthermore, regular fig consumption can also lower your risk of developing breast cancer, so is great for women who have a family history of this disease. Finally, figs contain a good dose of calcium per 8 oz serving, so they can help to boost bone strength in those who are at risk for osteoporosis.

46. GINGER

Ginger is a tasty spice that's a great addition to many different dishes, especially those that you are trying to create an Asian flare with. Ginger can help to reduce the level of gastrointestinal distress that you experience, and can also assist with the reduction of feelings of motion sickness, nausea, vomiting, and dizziness. In addition to that, ginger can help to enhance the overall health and function of your immune system, helping you feel healthier on an everyday basis. Especially for those leading active lifestyles, maintaining a strong immune system is important because this will help you recover faster from each workout that you perform.

47. GRAPES

Grapes are well-known for their flavonoid content and are also a terrific source of manganese, vitamin K, vitamin C, vitamin B1, as well as potassium. They're a powerful source of antioxidants that will help to defend against oxidative damage and help to prevent the onset of disease. In addition to that, regularly consuming grapes in your diet can also help to reduce the level of inflammation present in your body, assisting those who suffer from conditions such as arthritis. Finally, grapes will help to boost heart health by improving blood pressure levels, reducing the level of bad cholesterol in your body, decreasing the rate of LDL oxidation taking place in your system and making sure that you aren't experiencing red blood cells clumping together along the blood vessel lining. Grapes earn top marks for helping to ward off cardiovascular disease.

48. GREEK YOGURT, FAT FREE

Greek yogurt is going to be an excellent addition to your regular diet plan as it's high in calcium, low in sugar, and a good source of protein. While many dairy rich foods do need to be avoided by those who are suffering from GERD, if you choose lower fat varieties, they can be added to your diet plan. What's more is that foods that are high in dietary calcium tend to encourage faster abdominal fat loss, so by having these in the picture, you may just see faster results. Greek yogurt tastes great with some fresh berries, and topped with almonds or flaxseeds.

49. GREEN BEANS

Green beans make for a great side dish for many of the meals that you prepare throughout the week, and are quick to cook and add flavor to. Green beans will provide strong antioxidant support, reducing the rate of oxidation taking place in your body. In addition to that, green beans are also going to help boost your heart health, in part due to their omega-3 fat content. Green beans will reduce the level of inflammation present in the body, and lower the risk of developing diabetes. Just be sure to serve them up without the addition of butter so that you aren't adding saturated fat to this food.

50. HERBAL TEA

Herbal tea is a great beverage to drink for those who are suffering from GERD, as it's calorie free and, in some varieties, offers good health benefits as well. Coffee should be eliminated or reduced as much as possible if you're suffering from GERD, so herbal tea fits the bill well for something that you can drink instead. The hot beverage is a good choice for taking control of your hunger levels, as most people find the hot beverage rather soothing when they're suffering from high hunger levels. Serve some up with just a touch of honey if you need added sweetness, but avoid the overuse of sweetener products as these can do more harm than good as far as your health is concerned.

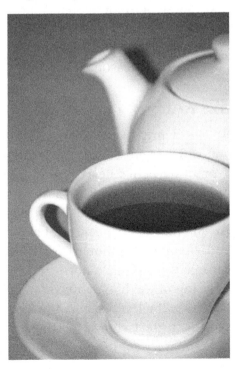

51. ICEBERG LETTUCE

Many people are very fast to assume that they should be avoiding any form of iceberg lettuce in their diet, as its commonly thought to be the lesser nutrient dense variety. While it is true that there are lettuce varieties that do come out slightly on top of iceberg lettuce, this variety isn't entirely devoid of nutrition either. Iceberg lettuce is going to provide you with thiamin, vitamin B6, iron, potassium, as well as vitamins C, A, and K. It'll also provide you with a small dose of folate, as well as manganese. Iceberg lettuce is incredibly low in calories, so it's a food that you can add into your diet without any concerns about weight gain at all, and appeals to many people for this reason.

52. KALE

Kale is a great vegetable to be adding to your diet if you suffer from GERD, and will go a long way towards promoting better heart health, as it's very effective for reducing your overall cholesterol level. In addition to that, kale is also a great source of vitamin K, vitamin A, vitamin C, manganese, fiber, tryptophan, calcium, and vitamin B6, amongst many other nutrients, so you can't go wrong from a nutritional point of view. Kale will offer top of the line antioxidant support, as well as help to reduce the level of inflammation present in the body, so it is a great choice for those who are experiencing inflammatory conditions. This leafy green vegetable may also help to lower your risk of bladder, breast, colon, or ovarian cancer, and will enhance your overall digestive system as well. Serve it up steamed to reap the most health benefits possible from this powerful food.

53. LEEKS

Leeks are a good vegetable to turn to if you're looking to maximize your cardiovascular system, as they'll help to protect your blood vessel linings from damage and oxidation. Additionally, they also increase the natural production of nitric oxide in the body, which can assist with the dilation and relaxation of blood vessels, enhancing overall heart function in the process. Leeks are also very rich in folate, so they are especially great for pregnant women to be consuming and may also help to reduce the risk of atherosclerosis, type 2 diabetes, as well as rheumatoid arthritis. Leeks work well steamed, added to soups, or just served alongside your main course meal.

54. LIMA BEANS

A bean that will quickly help you increase your dietary fiber consumption each day, lima beans are another great addition to your diet plan. This bean is rich in molybdenum, tryptophan, manganese, folate, potassium, iron and copper, and will also provide you with a good dose of vitamin B1. Eating lima beans on a regular basis may also assist with decreasing your risk of heart attack, due to their high dietary fiber content along with their high levels of folate and magnesium. This bean is rich in iron, which is important for ensuring proper red blood cell development, a key requirement for maintaining adequate energy levels. Finally lima beans, with their complex carbohydrate nature, are also going to be good at stabilizing your blood sugar levels, promoting a steady release of energy all day long. A must have food for any vegetarian, try this bean in a soup, chili, or just on its own next to your lean source of protein.

55. LENTILS

Lentils are another food that's very commonly consumed by vegetarians, and one that will make for a great addition to a GERD diet plan. Lentils are going to quickly absorb flavors of other foods they're paired next to, so they can be used in just about any dish that you happen to be preparing. Lentils are a good source of tryptophan, manganese, iron, phosphorus and copper in the diet, and will also provide you with some potassium. This makes them an ideal food for anyone who maintains an active lifestyle and who needs to keep their energy levels up. Finally, a study published in the Stroke Journal noted that they will help to reduce your risk of stroke as well.

56. MILLET

Millet works as a great replacement grain for brown rice in your diet plan, and can be used in just about any dish that you're making. It has a creamy taste, is enjoyed by many and will liven up any bland diet plan in a hurry. This food is rich in manganese content and is also going to offer a good dose of tryptophan, magnesium and phosphorus, all nutrients critical for promoting optimal health. This phosphorus found in millet will help to repair and rebuild damaged body tissues, making this food a must for anyone leading an active lifestyle. In addition to that, the magnesium content of millet is considerably higher than other foods, making it great for lowering your risk of type 2 diabetes. Furthermore, this grain can also help to lower the risk of gallstone development and help reduce the risk of breast cancer development as mentioned in a study in the International Journal of Epidemiology. As it is higher in calories like any grain, just be sure that you are measuring out your serving size so that you're eating an appropriate amount.

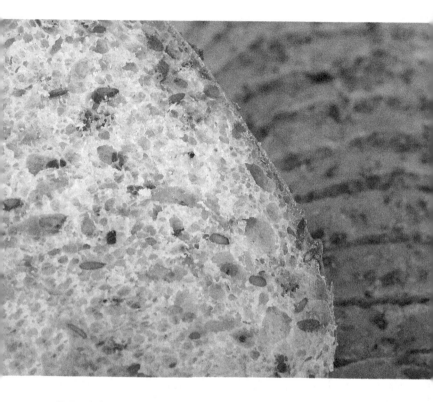

57. MULTI-GRAIN BREAD

Multi-grain bread is the route to take if you're going to be taking a sandwich to work for lunch, or starting your day off with a slice of toast smeared with almond butter. Multi-grain bread will contain a slower digesting source of complex carbohydrates that won't cause the blood glucose spike that white bread would, leaving you suffering from a blood sugar crash shortly thereafter.

Multi-grain bread will provide plenty of dietary fiber, helping to improve your heart health and lowering your risk of developing cardiovascular disease. In addition to that, multi-grain bread will also offer up a small dose of protein, so it can help you meet your daily needs if you're struggling. Just be sure that you do limit yourself to one or two slices per day as the carbohydrate calories still do add up. Also, avoid smearing butter or margarine over your multi-grain bread, as doing so will add unwanted fat and calories that will not help you maintain a healthy body weight.

58. MUSTARD GREENS

Mustard greens are a fantastic food for helping to lower your cholesterol levels, promoting optimal heart health. They're also going to help reduce the risk of cancer development due to their glucosinolate content, and are a very rich source of vitamin K, vitamin A, vitamin C, folate and manganese. Mustard greens are a good food to include in your diet if you want to cleanse and detoxify your system, ridding waste build-up that may have you feeling unwell. Finally, mustard greens can help to increase the overall level of circulation throughout the body, boosting heart health in this manner as well. Try them steamed for best health benefits, and served alongside your main protein source.

59. OATS

High in fiber, oats are a great cholesterol-reducing way to start your day off right. Complex carbohydrates such as oats are going to help to ensure that you maintain higher energy levels, keep your metabolic rate healthy and regulated, as well as help to improve recovery from intense workout sessions. Oatmeal is rich in manganese, selenium, phosphorus, magnesium and zinc, so it is a great food for improving the overall nutrition of your daily diet. Oats can also help to slow the progression of atherosclerosis in women past the age of menopause, and can boost overall immune system health and strength. Just be sure to purchase the plain variety so you aren't taking in added sugar with the oatmeal you eat. Add some cinnamon instead to enhance the flavor or consider adding a splash of almond milk for a creamier tasting dish.

60. OAT BRAN

If you want to boost your nutritional intake, one food that you must consider turning to is oat bran. Oat bran is very high in dietary fiber, so it will help to lower your cholesterol levels, improve heart health, regulate your blood glucose levels so that you don't experience energy highs and lows throughout the day, and help to prevent diabetes. Oat bran works perfect for baking, added on top of a bowl of oatmeal, or added to your protein shakes for a little additional dietary fiber. Oat bran is high in iron, protein, thiamin, magnesium, phosphorus, manganese and selenium. The iron content alone makes it a great choice for boosting your energy levels as you go about your day.

61. OREGANO

Oregano is a great spice to be adding to your diet plan and is high in vitamin K, manganese, iron, calcium and vitamin E. In addition to that, it's also very good for providing anti-bacterial effects in the body, reducing the risk that you fall ill due to infection, as mentioned in a study published in the Journal of Agricultural Food Chemistry. This spice is also very good for removing toxins from the colon, so it can help promote a healthier elimination system and reduce the risk of colon cancer. Finally, it can also help to lower the level of cholesterol in your body, enhancing your heart health dramatically. Those who are at risk of heart disease, or who have a family history of heart disease, will definitely want to make good use of this spice.

62. PARSNIPS

Parsnips are a good food to be adding to your diet when you need to break away from the common vegetables you're enjoying, and will offer numerous health benefits to your body. This vegetable is a great source of both types of fiber, insoluble as well as soluble, meaning it will work well to get your appetite under control and keep your bowels regular. It's also very high in vitamin C and contains folic acid, vitamin B6, thiamin, pantothenic acid and vitamin E. It'll also offer a small dose of iron, calcium, potassium, magnesium and phosphorus, and can help you regulate your blood pressure level. It is higher in sugar compared to some vegetables, so just be sure that you stay fully aware of this, and eat it in moderation.

63. PAPAYA

Papaya is a delicious fruit that's enjoyed by many on a seasonal basis, and offers a sweet taste that works great with many other foods. This fruit is loaded with vitamin C, providing over 313% of your total requirements. In addition to that, it's also a strong source of vitamin A, folate, potassium, and vitamins E and K. Papaya can be a great way to help stop heart disease before it starts, and will also help to reduce your risk of developing atherosclerosis. This fruit is great for reducing the level of cholesterol in the blood, and for lowering the chances of cholesterol build-up along the blood vessel walls leading to and from the heart. This fruit is going to enhance your overall digestive system health, and can reduce colon cancer by freeing your colon of toxic build-up. Finally, it's going to strengthen the immune system due to its combination of vitamins A and C, while providing anti-inflammatory effects, aiding those who suffer from asthma, osteoarthritis, and rheumatoid arthritis. Serve some up on its own or added into a fruit salad.

64. PEACHES

A peach is a perfect treat on any day when you're craving something sweet, and at only 68 calories per large peach, it's an easy add to just about any GERD diet plan. Peaches are a great source of fiber, and will also provide you with some vitamin A, niacin, potassium, as well as vitamin C. In addition to that, they'll help to strengthen your immune system and regulate heart as well as muscular contractions, making them a good addition to any active person's diet plan.

65. PEARS

Pears are one of the tastiest fruits that you could eat and offer a good dose of dietary fiber, ensuring that you maintain stable blood glucose levels while lowering your risk of cardiovascular disease. Pears are going to offer strong protection against free radicals due to their vitamin C and copper content, so they can help to kill bacteria and viruses that are invading your system before they contribute to you becoming ill. In addition to that, the copper found in pears can help to maintain proper white blood cell count and function, which is critical in maintaining a stronger immune system overall. Pears will also help to enhance your colon health due to their high fiber content, and may reduce your risk of developing colon cancer while also assisting women to ward off breast cancer development as noted by a study published in the International Journal of Cancer. Pears are great on

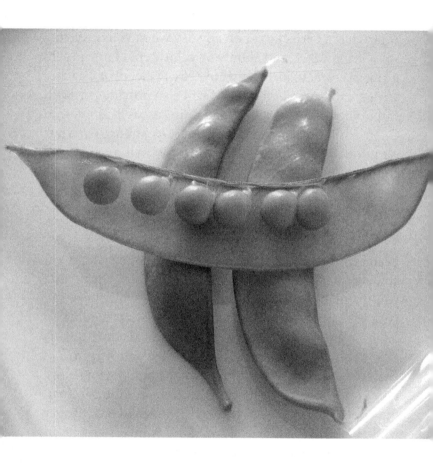

their own or added to a fruit salad. Just be sure to avoid canned pears, as they often come prepared in very high sugar syrups.

66. PEAS

For those who are picky eaters, peas are often a stand-by vegetable that they turn to. With a sweeter taste and ease of preparation, this vegetable works well with many different meals. Keep in mind that it is higher in calories than leafy greens, so you should moderate your serving size according to your calorie requirements. Peas are a fantastic source of vitamin K, manganese, vitamin C, vitamin B1, vitamin A, phosphorus, tryptophan, B vitamins, iron, copper, zinc, and potassium. All in all, they're a nutrient powerhouse that will help you maintain adequate energy levels, and support all the metabolic processes taking place in the body. Peas also supply antioxidant and anti-inflammatory benefits to the body, so by eating them regularly, you can help to reduce the risk of oxidation to your cells and help to enhance your overall health standing. Peas tend to help stabilize blood glucose levels as well, so they can be a good choice for those who are trying to defend against diabetes development.

67. PERCH

If you want a fat free source of high quality protein, look no further than to perch fish. This fish variety is an extremely clean variety to be eating, and is going to help to support your lean muscle mass building goals if you're leading an active lifestyle. If not, it'll simply help you meet your protein requirements with ease while consuming few calories in the process. Perch is a great source of niacin, vitamin B6, vitamin B12, calcium, and is also rich in phosphorus and selenium. Try it with some fresh steamed vegetables on the side, and drizzled with a small amount of olive oil for a complete meal that is sure to satisfy.

68. PINE NUTS

Pine nuts can be a great way to boost your healthy fat intake and get a little more protein in your day. Full of healthy fats, pine nuts will help to keep your blood sugar levels regulated while keeping your appetite down. This nut variety is high in fiber, contains no sugar, and is also a great source of thiamin. It'll also help to provide a good dose of manganese, and can work great tossed over a salad, added to muffins or pancakes, or just eaten on the side. If you're getting tired of constantly eating almonds or other nuts, give this nut a try instead.

69. POTATOES, BAKED

Potatoes are a commonly eaten, high-starch food that will supply you with plenty of energy as you go about your day. Potatoes are rich in vitamin C content, will provide a good dose of vitamin B6 and potassium, and can also help to boost your tryptophan intake. This vegetable also has a high phytochemical content, which allows it to be very effective for helping to ward off cardiovascular disease as well as respiratory conditions. A regular consumption of potatoes in your diet can also help to keep your blood pressure levels lower, boosting your heart health. Additionally, it can also help to promote a strong cardiovascular system and help increase the process of elimination from the body. Finally, the vitamin B6 found in potatoes can help to improve the usage of muscle glycogen during exercise, so this food earns top marks for boosting athletic performance as well.

70. PUMPKIN

Pumpkin is a delicious food that often goes overlooked in many people's diets, because they are so used to just eating it at Thanksgiving in the form of pumpkin pie. But, pumpkin can also be added into oatmeal, used to prepare muffins, cupcakes, or even cheesecakes. It works great as a replacement for the typical fat called for in these recipes, helping to retain the needed moisture to create these dishes. Pumpkin is a great source of vitamin E and will also provide you with magnesium, phosphorus, potassium, copper, vitamin A, vitamin C, vitamin K, iron, and magnesium. With seven grams of fiber per one cup serving, this food will help you manage your blood glucose levels.

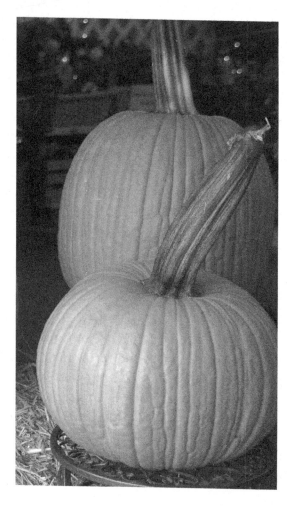

71. PRETZELS

If you're looking for a quick snack on the go, pretzels can be a good choice for those suffering from GERD. Since they are lower in fat content than many snack foods, this makes them a good choice for those who suffer from heartburn. Additionally, they'll supply you with a small amount of dietary fiber, which can help to ward off heart disease development. Just be sure that you are measuring out a single serving rather than eating them out of the bag because the calories can still add up if you aren't careful.

72. RADISHES

Radishes are a good food to consume if you're looking to boost the flavor of your dishes without adding many calories. This vegetable is used more as a condiment or garnish than a main component of the dish due to its potent taste, but offers good nutrition nevertheless. Radishes are a good source of riboflavin, vitamin B6, calcium, magnesium, copper, manganese and are also going to provide a small dose of vitamin C, folate and potassium. They tend to work best added to salads, however don't feel limited to using them just in these dishes. Add them wherever you feel they would taste great in the regular dishes you prepare for your diet plan.

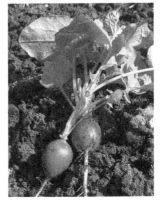

73. RICE, BROWN

Rice is a complex carbohydrate that will provide the body with a primary form of energy when added to your GERD diet plan. If you can always choose brown rice over white, as it's slightly less processed and contains more dietary fiber, along with other nutrients to support better overall health. Brown rice is rich in manganese, selenium, magnesium and tryptophan, and will provide strong antioxidant protection to the body as well. Brown rice, being that it is high in dietary fiber and selenium, can help to combat your risk of colon cancer, while also improving your thyroid function and possibly reducing your chances of a sluggish metabolism. This makes it a smart addition for anyone who is aiming to see weight loss results. Brown rice can assist with the lowering of cholesterol levels in the body, reducing your chances of coronary heart disease as noted by the American Journal of Clinical Nutrition, and will also provide help maintaining a proper blood pressure level. Finally, the magnesium found in brown rice will also help to regulate muscle contractions, so it is important for those who want to maintain an active lifestyle.

74. RICE CAKES

For a light snack throughout the day when you need something on the go, rice cakes can be a good option. They're low in fat and contain a small dose of dietary fiber, so they are a good option for those who are watching their body weight. They will provide a faster source of energy compared to some of the slower digesting carbohydrates you could eat, so they can work well as a pre-exercise snack when needed. If eating them throughout the day, try and combine them with a source of protein or healthy fats, such as almond butter or some canned tuna, to help reduce the release of the carbohydrates into the blood. As they come in many different flavors, you should easily be able to find one that will satisfy your taste buds.

75. ROMAINE LETTUCE

If you're looking to liven up your salads, one food that you must be sure you're getting is romaine lettuce. Romaine lettuce is a nutrition dense, leafy green that will help to keep your calorie intake down while still providing you top of the line nutrition. Romaine lettuce is rich in vitamin A, vitamin K, vitamin C, folate, fiber, manganese, potassium, iron, B vitamins and even a small amount of calcium. Romaine lettuce can help to decrease the formation of plaque in the artery walls, as well as lowering the risk of heart attacks or stroke. Try this leafy green in your salads as suggested, or in sandwiches, pitas, or on a lean ground beef or turkey burger.

76. RUTABAGA

Rutabagas are a vegetable that many people don't consume in their diet simply because they don't ever think about it, or they don't know how to prepare it in a delicious manner that will please their taste buds. But, if you experiment, you should be able to find a way to serve this that you'll enjoy. This vegetable is a great source of thiamin, vitamin B6, calcium, magnesium, phosphorus, vitamin C, potassium and manganese. It's a cholesterol free food, so it's good for those who are watching their heart health. Finally, the vitamin C content in this vegetable will help to strengthen the immune system so that you fall ill less frequently.

77. RYE BREAD

If you're looking for a hearty alternative to regular wheat bread, consider rye bread instead. This bread variety is an excellent choice for keeping your blood glucose levels stabilized, as it'll break down in the body more slowly than regular white or even whole wheat bread. In addition to that, it's also a great source of manganese, fiber, tryptophan and phosphorus, and will supply a small dose of magnesium. Rye bread can boost the level of satiety you feel after eating it, making it less likely that you snack in the hours following, and more likely that you follow your reduced calorie diet plan. In addition to that, it'll also help to reduce the formation of gallstones in the body while enhancing insulin sensitivity and warding off diabetes.

78. SEA VEGETABLES

Sea vegetables are a terrific source of iron in the diet, so they are important for those who don't consume a high volume of red meat but maintain an active exercise plan. Sea vegetables are also enriched with vitamin C, which can boost the iron absorption that occurs, and are also high in iodine, which promotes a healthy thyroid gland. These vegetables provide strong antioxidant protection to the body, so they are a vegetable that shouldn't be missed.

79. SESAME SEEDS

Sesame seeds are a great way to get in some healthy fats and are a good source of copper, manganese, tryptophan, calcium, magnesium, iron and phosphorus. Additionally, they're also rich in zinc and selenium, so they are great for males hoping to sustain their libido level. The copper content found in sesame seeds can help to provide some relief from symptoms of rheumatoid arthritis, and may boost the elasticity in the blood vessels, bones, as well as joints. Finally, the magne-sium found in this healthy fat will help to reduce the risk of asthma attack, lower blood pressure levels, and reduce the risk of heart attack, stroke and heart disease. Try some over salads or in your baked goods for added flavor.

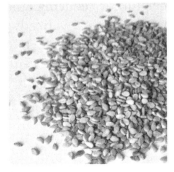

80. SKIM MILK

Skim milk is a good, low-fat source of calcium to be adding to your GERD diet plan and is a great way to promote strong bones. A cup of skim milk will also provide close to 10 grams of protein, making it ideal for those who are looking to boost their intake and meet their daily needs. Milk also contains CLA, which can help to reduce the risk of skin cancer while lowering your chances of developing atherosclerosis. Try some on its own, added to a fruit smoothie, or served with your morning bowl of cereal.

81. SPELT

Spelt is a terrific grain that has a nutty flavor and will provide you with a lasting source of energy that doesn't leave you hanging shortly after eating it. Spelt is high in manganese, fiber, phosphorus, vitamin B3, magnesium and copper and can help to lower your blood cholesterol levels, promoting a healthier heart. One study published in the American Heart Journal also noted that it's especially helpful for reducing atherosclerosis in postmenopausal women who are already suffering from coronary artery disease. In addition to this, regularly consuming this grain in your diet can assist with the prevention of gallstone development.

82. SPINACH

Spinach is a terrific leafy green to add to your diet and is especially high in iron and calcium content. Spinach is going to help you sustain higher energy levels, especially during intense physical activity, and will also help to boost your immune system. It has strong anti-inflammatory benefits and can assist with the reduction of cancer. Those who don't drink a high amount of milk in their diet will want to be sure to turn to spinach instead to help boost their bone strength and integrity. Try it in salads or added to a pita for lunch.

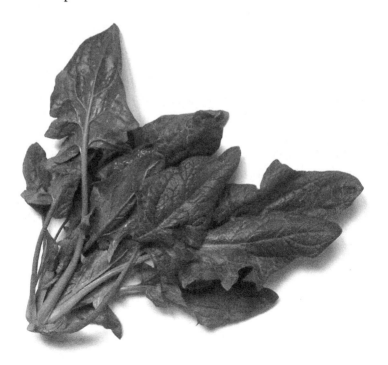

83. SORREL

Sorrel is a fast way to liven up any salad you're eating, as it's a sour-tasting green that will definitely offer a change of pace from the usual greens that you're likely used to. This green is very low in calories, containing just 15 per one cup serving, and will provide you with a good dose of fiber, vitamin C, along with iron to help maintain strong energy levels. Maintaining a diet high in iron is important so that you can keep your red blood cell count up, which transport oxygen to the working muscle cells.

84. SOYBEANS

Soybeans are a food that can be a good choice for vegetarians to help boost their protein intake while sticking to their diet. Soybeans provide a good source of vitamin K, folate, calcium, magnesium, as well as iron, all essential nutrients to support a healthy body. In addition to that, they're also very rich in antioxidant content, so they can assist with defending against oxidation and free radical damage in the body. Soybeans should be eaten sparingly among men, however, as the jury is still out on the long-term effects of high soy consumption on the male body.

85. SOY NUTS

Soy nuts are a good way to boost your healthy fat intake in your diet, and break away from the usual nut varieties that you're eating. A regular consumption of soy in the diet can help to lower overall cholesterol levels, so this can be a smart food to get into your plan. Soy nuts are rich in protein, contain some dietary fiber, and will also supply you with a good dose of folate, magnesium, riboflavin, as well as thiamin. Try them eaten on their own, toasted for added taste, or sprinkled over a salad instead.

86. SOY MILK

Soy milk can be a good alternative for those following a GERD diet plan who can't tolerate lactose found in cow's milk, or who simply prefer the taste of soy milk more. Soy milk is slightly higher in fat compared to skim milk, however it's a healthy fat so it can be part of your overall diet plan. Each one cup serving will provide just over 100 calories and 4 grams of protein, while being a good source of phosphorus as well as calcium.

87. STEAK, EXTRA LEAN, BROILED

Steak is a good way to get some high quality protein in and is rich in selenium, vitamin B3, zinc, vitamin B6, vitamin B12 as well as choline and phosphorus. Steak is rich in iron content especially, which is vital for making sure that you maintain high energy levels throughout the day, especially when exercising. Steak will also help to enhance your overall heart health due to its vitamin B6 and B12 content, and can also help to reduce the risk of colon cancer. Always choose the leanest varieties possible to minimize saturated fat intake.

88. STRAWBERRIES

Strawberries are an outstanding food for their vitamin C content, which will help to promote a strong immune system. In addition to that, they'll also help support heart health and can lower the level of inflammation in the body, while providing serious antioxidant support.

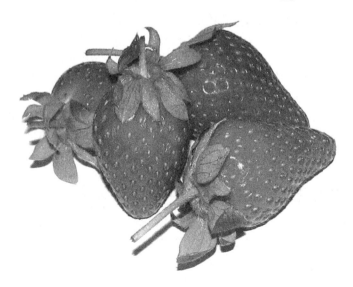

89. SQUASH

Squash is a great lower calorie food to have instead of mashed potatoes, and can be prepared in a number of different manners. Squash is high in fiber content and also rich in B vitamins for energy, as well as potassium to ensure proper muscular contractions. Those who eat squash on a regular basis can also assist with lowering their cholesterol levels.

90. SWEET BELL PEPPERS

Rich in antioxidants, sweet bell peppers are great for reducing your risk of cancer and defending against free radical damage. This food is high in both vitamin C and vitamin A, and will also provide multiple B vitamins. A regular consumption of bell peppers can help to reduce the harmful effects of inflammation, so is a great option by anyone suffering from inflammatory conditions. Finally, they can assist with promoting a healthy metabolism, as noted by a study published in the Amino Acids Journal.

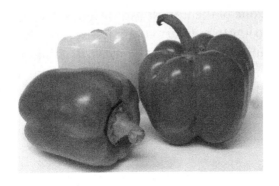

91. SWEET POTATOES

Sweet potatoes are the healthier alternative to regular potatoes, and are going to produce a slower increase in blood glucose levels while enhancing your dietary fiber intake. This vegetable is great baked, barbequed, or mashed, and offers a unique taste over the regular variety. It can help to lower your cholesterol levels, while enhancing energy levels throughout physical activity.

92. THYME

Want a low calorie way to flavor your foods? Try adding thyme. This spice works great with a number of different dishes and is a great source of vitamin K, iron, manganese, calcium and fiber. This spice also offers antioxidant protection and can support proper maintenance of cell membranes in the body, including those in the brain, kidney and heart cells.

93. TILAPIA

Tilapia is one of the leanest fish varieties that you can eat and is also low in mercury content, so it is safe to consume on a regular basis. This fish variety is going to provide a healthy dose of protein and is also high in selenium, which can help to boost the health of your brain. In addition to that, it provides a good dose of vitamin B12, which is important for maintaining a healthy metabolic rate.

94. TOFU

Tofu is a good alternative source of protein when you don't want to eat animal products, and is lower in saturated fat than many meats. Tofu provides a good source of calcium in the diet, and will also supply you with manganese, iron and omega-3 fats. This protein source is rich in selenium, copper, as well as phosphorus, and can boost your heart health. Finally, it may help to reduce the occurrence of cancer development, so it is a great option for anyone concerned about this disease.

95. TUNA

A great source of protein along with some omega fats, tuna is going to help to rebuild and repair body tissues while promoting a lean body composition. Tuna can be prepared a wide number of different ways, and has a flavor most people enjoy. It's a good source if thiamin, riboflavin, vitamin B6, phosphorus, vitamin A, niacin and vitamin B12.

96. TURNIP

Turnips can be a good alternative to serving up potatoes when you're trying to keep your calorie count down as they contain

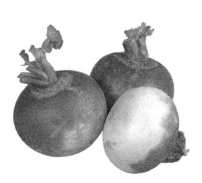

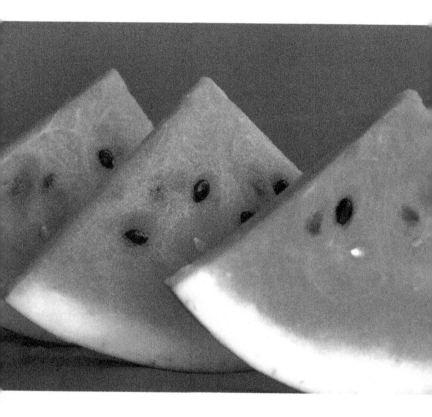

just 36 calories per cup. They are a fat free food and contain 2 grams of dietary fiber per serving, so they will help to control blood sugar levels while keeping your cholesterol levels down. They're also rich in calcium, potassium, copper and vitamin C.

97. WATERCRESS

If you'd like to change up your regular salad, consider adding watercress instead of your typical leaf variety. This leafy green contains just four calories per cup and is a great source of pantothenic acid, copper, vitamin A, vitamin C, vitamin E as well as thiamin and riboflavin. From a nutritional point of view, you definitely cannot go wrong with this choice. It'll support a strong immune system and help to decrease the levels of inflammation in the body.

98. WATERMELON

Watermelon is a juicy fruit that will help to keep you hydrated and also provide strong antioxidant protection at the same time. Watermelon is rich in lycopene, meaning it'll help to combat free radical damage and reduce the level of inflammation in the body. This fruit can also help to reduce your risk of prostate cancer as well as stroke.

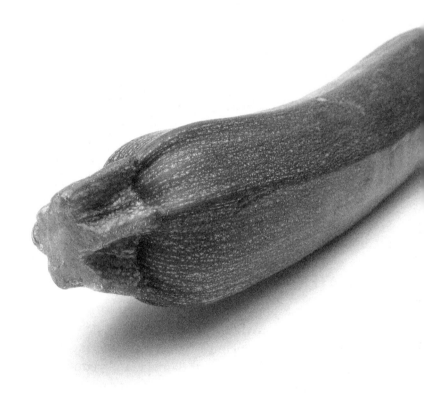

99. WHITE NAVY BEANS

Navy beans are a great way to boost the fiber content in your diet and provide a long-lasting source of energy that won't quit. They're rich in folate, tryptophan, manganese, and vitamin B1, and will also offer some protein to your diet. Rich in iron, this bean will help you finish your workouts without feeling fatigued. Great for lowering cholesterol, try adding them to a chili or as a side dish.

100. YAMS

Yams are another good alternative to the regular potato and will help to lower cholesterol levels, increase your dietary fiber intake, and help promote a healthier heart. Since they will assist in keeping blood glucose levels stable, they're also great for helping to ward off diabetes development. Try them baked or mashed for great flavor.

101. ZUCCHINI

Zucchini is a delicious vegetable that works great in salads, on its own, baked, or grilled and is a good source of thiamin, niacin, pantothenic acid, vitamin A, vitamin C and vitamin B6. In addition to that, it's also rich in folate, magnesium, phosphorus and zinc. Serve some up when you need a change from the everyday vegetables you're consuming.

CONCLUSION

So there you have 101 great foods to add to your GERD diet plan. If you create a healthy meal plan in advance using primarily these foods, you can feel confident that you're doing what you can to maximize the health benefits you derive from your meals, while maintaining control over your symptoms.

While it may take a little more effort on your part to put together a sound menu, it's well worth it when you see the difference it makes in how you feel on a day to day basis.

New medical study reported by Fox News warns that stomach acid drugs can kill! Check out this Kitchen Cure for Acid Reflux... CureGERD.info

Handy List for Shopping for the 101 Best Foods To Treat and Cure GERD

Below you will find the foods listed in a section where you might find them in a grocery store. Some items may be found in more than one place in your store, so that is why you will find them listed in more than one section below.

Whenever possible ... eat FRESH ... not canned or preserved. Enjoy!

FRESH PRODUCE

Apples

Apricots

Artichokes

Asparagus

Avocado

Bananas

Basil

Beets

Blackberries

Black current

Blueberries

Bok Choy

Broccoli

Brussels sprouts

Butter lettuce

Cabbage

Cantaloupe

Carrots

Celery

Cherries

Chives

Cilantro

Coconut

Cucumber

Endive

Eggplant

Figs

Ginger

Grapes

Green beans

Iceberg lettuce

Kale

Leeks

Lima beans

Mustard greens

Oregano

Parsnips

Papaya

Peaches

Pears

Peas

Potatoes, baked

Pumpkin

Radishes

Romaine lettuce

Rutabaga

Sea vegetables

Spinach

Sorrel

Soybeans

Strawberries

Squash

Sweet bell peppers

Sweet potatoes

Thyme

Turnip

Watercress

Watermelon

Yams

Zucchini

NUTS/SEEDS

Almonds

Pine nuts

Sesame seeds

Soy nuts

MEAT/FISH

Beef, ground, extra lean

Chicken breast, skinless

Cod

Perch

Steak, extra lean, broiled

Tilapia

Tuna

REFRIGERATED / DAIRY CASE

Almond milk

Cream cheese, fat free

Egg whites

Feta Cheese, low fat

Greek yogurt, fat free

Skim milk

Soy milk

Tofu

LENTILS/GRAINS

Black beans

Lentils

Rice, white or brown

White navy beans

Lima beans

BAKING/STAPLES

Almond butter

Cayenne pepper

Basil

Ginger

Oregano

Thyme

DRINK

Chamomile tea

Herbal tea

CANNED VEGETABLES

Applesauce, unsweetened

Artichokes

Black beans

Beets

Carrots

Green beans

Peas

Pumpkin

HEALTH FOOD SECTION/STORE

Almond milk

Acai berry

Alfalfa

Buckwheat

Spelt

Tofu

FROZEN CASE

Broccoli

Brussels sprouts

Carrots

Green beans

Lima beans

Peaches

Peas

Spinach

Strawberries

CEREAL/RICE /PASTA

Bran cereal

Corn bran cereal

Millet

Oats

Oat bran

DRIED FRUIT

Black current

Apricots

Blackberries

Cherries

Figs

BREAD SECTION

Multi-grain bread

Rye bread

MISC.

Pretzels

Rice cakes

"NEW STUDY WARNS: STOMACH ACID DRUGS CAN KILL"

This Natural Remedy Puts Out The Fire Of Stomach Acid Pain And Acid Reflux - Safe, Cheap, Effective Relief

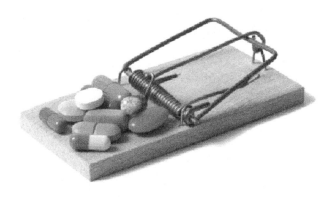

A new study says the drugs you take for acid reflux and excess stomach acid may be worse than the disease itself.

In fact, treating acid reflux with these drugs has now been linked to an early death.

The study, published in a recent edition of the journal *Clinical Infectious Diseases,* concludes that stomach acid plays a crucial role in stopping infections in the body.

The problem?

According to Fox News, **"medications that suppress**

the production of stomach acid... make people more susceptible to complications of gastrointestinal infections, including **raising the risk of dying."**

The study's author, Dr. Edith R. Lederman, is an infectious disease specialist at the Naval Medical Center in San Diego.

Dr. Lederman says "this is the first study to have found an **association between use of antacids and increase of mortality."**

While this raises some **very serious concerns** for stomach acid sufferers, there is **some good news...**

NATURAL METHODS STILL THE SAFEST BET... AND VERY EFFECTIVE

You can finally put that fire out in your chest with cheap, safe, and natural remedies.

Because for twenty years I've studied the experiments, and results of leading researchers in the area of what I call "refluxology" and discovered **simple natural remedies for heartburn and acid reflux** that work 100% of the time for nearly everyone who uses them.

In fact, my discoveries have relieved the symptoms of **acid reflux for people** all around the world...AND helped them kick the acid reflux "drug habit" for good . . . completely avoid surgery . . . and enjoy the foods they love without fear.

The best news is, this approach is so easy and inexpensive that you can get **everything you need to control your heartburn and acid reflux forever** at the local grocery store and **for less than ten dollars.**

NATURAL CURES ENDORSED BY MEDICAL DOCTORS

A handful of doctors are getting behind the push to educate patients about what really works to snuff their acid reflux symptoms naturally.

Dr. Scott Saunders. M.D., says natural approaches are the key. **"Studying natural medicine is power,"** he says, explaining that **you can absolutely treat your acid reflux yourself** with simple steps that...

→ Are fast, painless, safe, and natural

→ Based on proven home remedies

→ Have zero negative side effects

→ Will help you save thousands of dollars in medical bills, drugs, and hospital stays

→ Will free you from stress and fear of infections

→ Will improve your overall health and immune system

If you suffer from acid reflux, you cannot afford to ignore the truth about how to avoid the dangerous side effects of stomach acid drugs. Side effects like the ones described in the latest study - including premature death.

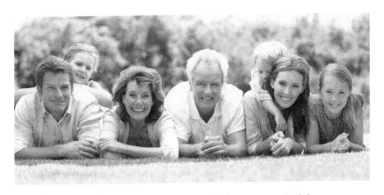

Make sure you're there to watch your children grow up...enjoy life far into your golden years with the ones you love. Go here before you pop another life-threatening pill: CureGERD.info

But the good news is you don't have to let that happen. And you definitely don't have to rely on expensive, dangerous drugs that don't work! You can find out how to **relieve your own acid reflux** and stomach acid problems when you **watch a FREE, informative presentation**, and see how to fix the real cause of your excess stomach acid... using **natural, safe, and easy methods that are virtually free.**

Now you can **protect yourself** with cutting-edge information on **healing yourself** or your loved ones of excess stomach acid, painful heartburn, and acid reflux. **Watch this free video** and discover **how to control your acid reflux safely, once and for all.**

CureGERD.info

REFERENCES:

Appel LJ, Moore TJ, Obarzanek E, et al.A clinical trial of the effects of dietary patterns on blood pressure. DASH Collaborative Research Group. N Engl J Med. 1997 Apr 17;336(16):1117-24. 1997.

Augustsson K, Michaud DS, Rimm EB, et al. A prospective study of intake of fish and marine fatty acids and prostate cancer. Cancer Epidemiol Biomarkers Prev. 2003 May;12(1)64-7. 2003. PMID:12540506.

Bazzano LA, He J, Odgen LG et al. Dietary intake of folate and risk of stroke in US men and women:NHANES I Epidemiologic Follow-up Study. Stroke 2002 May;33(5):1183-9. 2002.

Cade JE, Burley VJ, Greenwood DC.Dietary fibre and risk of breast cancer in the UK Women's Cohort Study. Int J Epidemiol. 2007 Jan 24; [Epub ahead of print] . 2007. PMID:17251246.

Calucci L, Pinzino C, Zandomeneghi M et al. Effects of gamma-irradiation on the free radical and antioxidant contents in nine aromatic herbs and spices. J Agric Food Chem 2003 Feb 12; 51(4):927-34. 2003.

Cooper AJL, Krasnikov BF, Niatsetskaya ZV et al. Cysteine S-conjugate β-lyases: Important roles in the metabolism of naturally occurring sulfur and selenium-containing compounds, xenobiotics and anticancer agents. Amino Acids. 2011 June; 41(1): 7–27. 2011.

Erkkila AT, Herrington DM, Mozaffarian D, Lichtenstein AH. Cereal fiber and whole-grain intake are associated with reduced progression of coronary-artery atherosclerosis in postmenopausal women with coronary artery disease. Am Heart J. 2005 Jul;150(1):94-101. 2005.

Jensen MK, Koh-Banerjee P, Hu FB, Franz M, Sampson L, Gronbaek M, Rimm EB. Intakes of whole grains, bran, and germ and the risk of coronary heart disease in men. Am J Clin Nutr 2004 Dec;80(6):1492-9. 2004.

Mathews JN, Flatt PR, and Abdel-Wahab YH. Asparagus adscendens (Shweta musali) stimulates insulin secretion, insulin action and inhibits starch digestion. The British Journal of Nutrition. Cambridge: Mar 2006. Vol. 95, Iss. 3; p. 576-581. 2006.

Rios JL, Recio MC, Escandell JM, et al. Inhibition of transcription factors by plant-derived compounds and their implications in inflammation and cancer. Curr Pharm Des. 2009;15(11):1212-37. Review. 2009.

Suzuki R, Rylander-Rudqvist T, Ye W, et al. Dietary fiber intake and risk of postmenopausal breast cancer defined by estrogen and progesterone receptor status--a prospective cohort study among Swedish women. Int J Cancer. 2008 Jan 15;122(2):403-12. 2008. PMID:17764112.

Zheng W, Wang SY. Antioxidant activity and phenolic compounds in selected herbs. J Agric Food Chem 2002;49:5165-70. 2002.

Made in the USA
Las Vegas, NV
15 June 2022